PRESERVATION AND CANNING OF VEGETABLES

Developing the Skill of Canning and Preserving Vegetables

Islamiyyah Fasasi

COPYRIGHT

TABLE OF CONTENTS

INTRODUCTION

The technique of preserving vegetables to increase their shelf life while retaining their nutritional value, flavor, and quality is known as vegetable preservation. It is a centuries-old method that has changed throughout time as technology and our knowledge of food science have advanced. By preventing food waste and spoiling, preservation techniques enable people to enjoy seasonal produce all year round, especially in places where specific veggies might not be easily accessible. Vegetable preservation is crucial for maintaining food security as well as extending the shelf life of fresh vegetables, particularly in areas where agriculture may be seasonal or subject to weather-related disturbances. Households can also save money by purchasing in bulk during busy seasons and conserving extra produce for later use.

Vegetables can be preserved in several ways, including canning, freezing, drying, pickling, and fermenting. Every technique has special benefits and can be customized to fit the tastes and needs of various vegetable varieties. For instance, freezing works well for veggies that are sensitive to high temperatures, like peas and maize, while canning is best for low-acid crops, like carrots and green beans

CHAPTER ONE

Knowing the Fundamentals of Canning

Principles of Canning

The technique of heat processing is used in canning to eradicate any bacteria, yeasts, or mold that may be present in vegetables. Vegetables can be securely preserved at room temperature for extended periods by sealing the jars and exposing them to high temperatures, which eliminates hazardous germs.

Two main canning techniques are frequently used: pressure canning and water bath canning. While pressure canning is required for low-acid vegetables like beans and corn, water bath canning is appropriate for high-acid vegetables like tomatoes and pickles.

- Water Bath Canning: This process entails immersing packed jars of acidic vegetables in boiling water for a predetermined amount of time. In addition to eliminating microbes, the heat produces a vacuum seal that keeps food from spoiling. Water bath canning is a great method for preserving vegetables, such as tomatoes, pickles, and fruit jams.

- Pressure Canning: Low-acid crops like beans, corn, and potatoes require pressure canning, as opposed to water bath canning. Boiling water is insufficient to destroy dangerous germs from these veggies; higher temperatures are needed. Precise temperature and pressure control are made possible with a pressure canner, guaranteeing secure preservation.

Safety Measures

When it comes to canning veggies, safety is crucial. Equipment such as jars, lids, and utensils should be properly sterilized to help avoid contamination and spoiling. Vegetables can be safely canned at the right temperatures and processing periods if you use tried-and-true recipes from reputable sources like the USDA or the National Center for Home Food Preservation.

Additionally, it is imperative to utilize fresh, premium products free of flaws or decay indicators and to check veggies for symptoms of rotting before canning. Vegetables that are canned should be kept out of direct sunlight and kept in a cool, dark place to preserve their quality and shelf life.

Equipments needed

A few key items of equipment are needed to begin canning vegetables at home, including:

- Jars for canning with bands and lids
- Pressure canners or water bath canners
- Funnel for canning
- Jar raiser
- Tool for removing bubbles
- A timer for the kitchen
- A food thermometer

Purchasing top-notch equipment makes successful canning operations safe and feasible while also enabling effective and pleasurable at-home food preservation.

Successful vegetable preservation starts with a thorough understanding of canning fundamentals. People can gain great satisfaction from stocking their cupboards with wholesome and tasty canned veggies that they can eat all year long by taking the necessary safety steps, sticking to tried-and-true recipes, and utilizing the right tools.

CHAPTER TWO

Selection of Vegetables for Canning

High-Acid Vegetables

- Examples: Pickles, peppers, tomatoes, and most fruits.

- Suitable Method: Water bath canning.

- Why They Work: Because high acidity levels prevent hazardous bacteria from growing, high-acid fruits and vegetables can be safely canned using the water bath process. Using this approach, prepared veggies are preserved for long-term storage by immersing jars of them in boiling water for a predetermined amount of time.

Low-Acid Vegetables

- Examples: Potatoes, carrots, peas, maize, and green beans.

- Suitable Method: Pressure canning.

- Why They Work: Pressure canning's greater temperatures and pressures are necessary for the safe preservation of low-acid vegetables. These veggies might contain dangerous bacteria like Clostridium botulinum, which if eaten, can result in botulism poisoning if they are not properly processed.

Ripeness and Freshness

Select produce that is in season, ripe, and devoid of defects or decaying elements. When canned, vegetables that are at the height of their ripeness produce the finest flavor and texture. Steer clear of overripe or underripe food since it may not keep well and may degrade the finished product.

Taste and Texture

When choosing which vegetables to can, pay attention to their flavor and texture. Certain veggies work best when they are crisp and tender, such as cucumbers for pickling or green beans for canning. Others, like tomatoes for soups or sauces, could be better off when they are ripe and tender.

Preparation Requirements

Before canning, consider the preparation needs of various veggies. While some veggies can be canned whole or chopped, others may need to be blanched, peeled, or sliced. Select veggies based on your level of experience and available time for preparation.

Seasons & Accessibility

Take advantage of the bounty of the season when choosing veggies to can. The highest flavor and nutritional content are guaranteed in the finished product when veggies are canned while they are at their freshest. Furthermore, take into account the vegetables that are available in your area and select ones that are both reasonably priced and easily obtainable.

Personal References and Recipes

When choosing veggies for canning, take your tastes and the recipes you want to utilize into account. To get the best results, select the vegetables that work best with the recipes or flavor combinations you want to use.

Dietary restrictions and family preferences

When choosing veggies for canning, consider your family members' nutritional requirements and preferences. When selecting veggies and recipes, take into account any allergies, intolerances, or preferences. Prioritize preserving veggies that your family loves and eats on a daily basis.

CHAPTER THREE

Methods of Preservation

Canning

Berries, tomatoes, pickles, and other high-acid produce can all be preserved using the water bath canning method. To make a vacuum seal, vegetables are placed into jars, covered with a liquid (such as syrup or vinegar), and then placed in boiling water for a predetermined amount of time.

Pressure Canning: To properly preserve low-acid crops like corn, carrots, and green beans, pressure canning is necessary. The jars and their contents are heated to a high temperature in a pressure canner, which eliminates dangerous microorganisms and guarantees secure long-term preservation.

Freezing

Vegetables can be preserved easily and effectively by freezing them. Vegetables are quickly cooled in ice water and frozen after a brief blanch in hot water. Vegetables can be frozen for several months and their flavor and nutrients are preserved. They work well in casseroles, stir-fries, and soups.

Desiccating (drying)

By taking out the moisture from vegetables, dehydration prevents the formation of mold and bacteria. You can dry vegetables in an oven, dehydrator, or even outside in the sun. Dehydrated vegetables have a lengthy shelf life and need little space and weight. To use them in soups, stews, and snacks, simply rehydrate them.

Pickling

Pickling is the process of preserving vegetables in a vinegar, sugar, salt, and spice mixture. Because of this acidic environment's ability to prevent bacterial growth, vegetables can be safely kept at room temperature. Cucumbers, carrots, and peppers are examples of pickled vegetables that acquire acidic flavors and crunchy textures that go well with a wide range of foods.

Fermentation

Vegetable sugars and starches are converted into lactic acid by fermentation, a traditional preservation technique that uses beneficial bacteria to create an acidic environment that keeps food from spoiling. In addition to being preserved, fermented foods like pickles, kimchi, and sauerkraut also acquire rich tastes and probiotic advantages.

Root Cellaring

Vegetables are stored through the process of root cellaring in a cool, dark, and humid space, like a basement or root cellar. By creating ideal storage conditions that delay aging and stop sprouting and spoiling, this age-old method of preservation increases the shelf life of root vegetables such as potatoes, carrots, and beets.

CHAPTER FOUR

Canning Vegetables

Prepare your Workspace

Make sure your desk is tidy and orderly first. After giving yourself a good cleaning, collect all the supplies you will need, such as canning funnels, lids, bands, canning pots or pressure canners, jar lifters, and jars.

Select and Prepare your Vegetables

Select vegetables that are at their full ripeness and are of great quality. After giving them a thorough wash under running water, give them a trim or peel as needed. To guarantee equal cooking, chop the veggies into uniform pieces before putting them in jars.

Sterilize the Jars and Lids

Rinse the canning jars, lids, and bands thoroughly after washing them in hot, soapy water. Use your dishwasher's sanitize cycle or boil the jars and lids for ten minutes to sterilize them. Until the time comes to fill them, keep the jars and lids hot.

Fill your Jars

Pack the prepped veggies firmly into the sterilized jars, leaving the necessary headspace at the top, using a canning funnel. You can use a bubble remover tool or gently tap the jars on the tabletop to get rid of any air bubbles.

Apply Bands and Lids

To get rid of any food residue, use a clean, moist cloth to wipe the rims of the filled jars. After putting the jar lids on, tighten the bands with a fingertip's worth of force. To prevent tampering with the sealing process, do not over-tighten the bands.

Process your Jars

Fill the water bath canner with enough boiling water to cover the filled jars by at least one inch. This is known as water bath canning. As directed by your recipe and the altitude, process the jars for the specified amount of time.

Pressure Canning: Pack the filled jars into a pressure canner and process them by the pressure and time specified by the manufacturer for your recipe and altitude, as well as your recipe's instructions.

Cool and Check Seals

Once processing is finished, carefully take the jars out of the canner and set them on a cooling rack or fresh cloth to finish chilling. A popping sound should be audible as the jars cool, signifying that the lids have shut tightly. Apply pressure to the middle of each lid to inspect the seals. The jar seals if it does not flex or pop.

Label and Store your Jars

Using a permanent marker, write the contents and the canning date on each jar. The sealed jars should be kept out of direct sunlight and extremely hot or cold. A pantry or cellar would be a good place to store them. Vegetables that have been properly canned can be kept for a year or more.

CHAPTER FIVE

Storing Canned Vegetables

Inspection and Cooling

Allow the jars to cool completely at room temperature after the canning process is finished. After the jars have cooled, check them for any anomalies, such as bulging lids or leaks. If any jars appear to be spoiled, throw them away.

Labeling

Using a permanent pen or labels, write the contents and the canning date on each jar. When you label your jars properly, you can keep track of what is in each one and make sure that you rotate your stock for freshness by using the oldest jars first.

Storage Location

Vegetables canned in their sealed jars should be kept in a dry, dark, and cool place, like a pantry, cellar, or cupboard. Vegetables may deteriorate more quickly if they are exposed to heat, dampness, and direct sunshine.

Temperature Control

The ideal range for storage temperature is 50°F to 70°F (10°C to 21°C). Vegetables should not be kept in regions with large temperature swings, such as a garage without heat or close to heating vents. Establishment:

Place the jars carefully on racks or shelves, making sure there is enough room between each one and that they are not crammed too close together. This facilitates appropriate air circulation and facilitates jar access as needed.

Avoid Stacking

Although stacking jars to save space could be appealing, do not do so as this increases the chance of seal failure and puts excessive strain on the lids. To avoid breakage, store jars in a single layer instead.

Rotation

When utilizing your canned vegetables, rotate them according to the principle of FIFO (first in, first out). To make sure that nothing goes to waste from your canned goods, start with the oldest jars. For best quality, use the vegetables within the suggested timeframe and keep an eye out for expiration dates.

Monitoring

Check your canned vegetables for spoiling regularly. Look for things like bulging lids, strange coloring, or offensive smells. To avoid contamination, throw away the impacted jars right away if you find any anomalies.

CHAPTER SIX

Safety and Quality Assurance in Canning Vegetables

Follow Approved Recipes

Utilize only tried-and-true canning recipes from reputable sources like the National Center for Home Food Preservation or the United States Department of Agriculture. The processing times and ingredient amounts in these recipes have been verified by science.

Sanitation and Sterilization

Throughout the canning process, give cleanliness a priority. Before handling produce and tools, properly wash your hands, utensils, and work surfaces. Before using, sterilize canning jar lids, bands, and other components to get rid of dangerous bacteria and stop contamination.

Proper Processing Methods

Considering the acidity of the vegetables to be preserved, select the proper canning procedure. High-acid vegetables can be preserved safely by water bath canning, but low-acid veggies must be pressure-canning to achieve the required temperatures.

Keeping an Eye on Temperatures and Processing times.

Respect the suggested processing times and temperatures listed in authorized canning recipes to the letter. While overprocessing might cause the veggies to lose their texture and quality, underprocessing can allow dangerous bacteria to survive.

Examining the Integrity of the Seal

Check each jar for a proper seal after processing. Concave and strong to the touch, a sealed lid is what you want. Jars with damaged seals should be thrown away since they can be contaminated or have not been processed properly.

Storage Conditions

To ensure their quality and safety, store canned veggies in a cold, dark, and dry environment. Jars should not be kept in locations that are subject to extremes in temperature, direct sunshine, or high humidity since these elements might weaken the seals and cause deterioration.

Rotation and Regular Inspection

Check canned veggies that have been stored for signs of spoiling, such as bulging lids, strange coloring, or unpleasant smells, regularly. To avoid waste, rotate your jars according to the principle of "first in, first out," using the oldest jars first.

Education and Training

By participating in online courses, reading credible publications, or attending seminars, you may stay up to date on the latest advancements and best practices in food preservation. You may be sure that you stay current on vegetable canning safety procedures and methods by participating in ongoing education.

Quality Assurance

To get excellent results from your canning process, try to be consistent in your methods. Consider elements like the quality of the ingredients, how they are prepared, and how they are processed to create canned vegetables that are both wholesome and tasty.

CHAPTER SEVEN

Recipes and Ideas for Canned Vegetables

Classic Dill Pickles

Can cucumbers with garlic, dill, vinegar, and spices to make your crunchy dill pickles. Savor them as a refreshing snack, a topping for sandwiches, or a garnish for charcuterie boards.

Spicy Pickled Green Beans

Pickled green beans add a kick of spice to canned vegetables. For a tangy and tasty treat, pack blanched green beans into jars along with garlic, red pepper flakes, and a vinegar-based brine.

Tomato Sauce

Can homemade tomato sauce as a way to preserve the bounty of the summer. When thick and rich, simmer ripe tomatoes with onions, garlic, herbs, and a small amount of sugar. Once done, put in jars for easy use in soups, pizzas, and pasta dishes.

Salsa Verde

Revel in the vibrant tastes of green chiles and tomatillos with a zesty salsa verde. Puree roasted tomatillos, jalapeños, onions, cilantro, and lime juice; can the salsa to create a flexible sauce that goes well with tacos, enchiladas, and tortilla chips.

Carrot Ginger Soup Base

Pureed carrots combined with fresh ginger, onions, and vegetable broth can be canned to create a tasty soup foundation. Just warm up and serve for a nourishing and warming soup on chilly days.

Sweet Corn Relish

Save the summer corn's sweetness by preserving a tart corn relish. To make a versatile relish that goes great with grilled meats, sandwiches, and salads, combine corn kernels with bell peppers, onions, vinegar, sugar, and spices.

Zesty Giardiniera

Can a variety of pickled vegetables, such as bell peppers, celery, carrots, and cauliflower, to make your giardiniera. Combine oregano, garlic, and chili flakes to create a delicious sauce that goes well with salads and sandwiches.

Canned Pumpkin Puree

Can cook and mash pumpkin to stock your cupboard with homemade puree. All year round, use the puree to make pies, muffins, soups, and other seasonal dishes.

Mixed Vegetable Medley

Can a range of veggies, such as carrots, green beans, peas, and corn, to make a vibrant and nourishing mixed vegetable medley. For extra taste, season with garlic, herbs, and a small amount of vinegar.

Pickled Beet Salad

Beets can be preserved in a tart and sweet brine to make a tasty pickled beet salad. For a savory and colorful salad, serve the pickled beets with goat cheese, arugula, and walnuts.

CHAPTER EIGHT

Troubleshooting and Frequently Asked Questions (FAQ) for Canning Vegetables.

1. Problem: Jars Didn't Seal Properly

- Solution: Check for any nicks, cracks, or uneven rim surfaces on the jars. Make sure the lids and bands are clean and properly applied. If jars still fail to seal, refrigerate the contents and consume them within a few days, or reprocess with new lids.

2. Problem: Cloudy Liquid in Jars

- Solution: Cloudiness can result from minerals in the water used for canning or from starches released by overcooking vegetables. Using distilled or filtered water and avoiding overcooking can help prevent cloudiness. Cloudiness is usually safe to consume but may affect the appearance.

3. Problem: Vegetables Are Mushy

- Solution: Overcooking can cause vegetables to become mushy. Follow recommended processing times and avoid overcooking vegetables before canning. Choose firmer varieties of vegetables and blanch them briefly before canning to help retain texture.

4. Problem: Floating Vegetables in Jars

- Solution: Floating vegetables can occur if air pockets are trapped during packing or if the vegetables are not properly blanched before canning. Tap the jars gently on the countertop to remove air bubbles before sealing. Ensure vegetables are packed tightly and blanched as directed.

5. Problem: Distasteful Odor or Taste

- Solution: Tastes or smells off could be signs of spoiling from contamination or incorrect preparation. In the future, make sure that the right procedures for sterilization, processing, and storage are followed, and throw away any jars that have unpleasant tastes or smells.

6. Frequently Asked Question: Is It Possible to Reuse Canning Lids?

- Answer: Reusing canning lids is not advised, to answer your question. Lid sealing compound is intended for one-time use only; reusing it may result in an unreliable seal. To guarantee correct sealing, always use fresh, unused lids for every canning session.

7. Frequently Asked Question: What Is the Shelf Life of Canned Vegetables?

- Answer: When kept in a cold, dry, and dark place, canned veggies can survive up to a year or more. Before eating, it is crucial to examine the contents for symptoms of deterioration and to verify the seals.

8. Frequently Asked Question: Are Canning Recipes Adjustable?

- Answer: It is not advised to modify canning recipes by

changing the amounts of ingredients or the way they are processed. Use tried-and-true recipes from reputable sources to guarantee quality and safety.

9. Frequently Asked Question: Is It Possible to Can My Own Vegetables?

- Answer: Vegetables from your garden can indeed be canned. To guarantee safe preservation, it is crucial to use high-quality, fresh food, adhere to suggested processing procedures, and maintain good hygiene standards.

10. Frequently Asked Question: Is It Possible to Freeze Vegetables?

- Answer:Vegetables should not be frozen after canning. The jars may break or crack as a result of freezing, jeopardizing the seal and perhaps causing spoiling. Instead, keep canned vegetables in a dry, dark, and cool place.

CONCLUSION

Vegetable canning is a culinary technique that enables you can preserve the flavors and freshness of the harvest season all year long, not just a means of preservation. Vegetables that have been canned offer convenience and diversity to your cupboard, delivering a hint of summer in every bite, from crunchy pickles to flavorful tomato sauces.

We have covered all the essentials of vegetable preservation in this extensive book, from comprehending canning concepts to becoming proficient with sophisticated methods. Everything from choosing the freshest produce to resolving common problems and providing answers to frequently asked queries has been covered.

You can confidently start your canning journey by adhering to recommended canning procedures, placing a high priority on safety and quality assurance, and encouraging creativity in your recipe development and taste combinations. In the realm of vegetable canning, there is always something new to learn and uncover, regardless of your experience level.

Therefore, prepare for a gastronomic adventure by rolling up your sleeves, gathering your equipment, and letting your imagination run wild as you preserve vegetables. Your reward for your hard work, attention to detail, and creative spirit will be jars full of colorful, nutrient-dense veggies that will add color to your meals and satisfy your palate for months to come. Cheers to canning!